The Scarsdale Diet Book

A Quick and Effective Way to Lose Weight and Improve Your Health

By

Nancy spicer

This book is a work of nonfiction and is intended for informational purposes only. The views expressed in this book are those of the author and do not necessarily reflect the official policies or positions of any other person, organization, or entity.

This book is not intended to provide legal, financial, or professional advice, and should not be used as such. The author and publisher shall not be liable for any loss or damages resulting from the use of the information contained in this book.

Table of contents

Introduction to the Scarsdale Diet

Kayla had always struggled with her weight. She had tried every diet out there, but nothing seemed to work. She was tired of feeling self-conscious and unhappy with her appearance. One day, she stumbled upon the Scarsdale Diet online. It promised quick and effective weight loss, and she was intrigued.

She decided to give it a try and started following the strict meal plan. It was tough at first, but she was determined to make it work. She cut out all processed and sugary foods and stuck to the recommended portion sizes. She also increased her water intake and started exercising regularly.

As the days went by, Kayla noticed that her clothes were fitting looser and she was starting to feel more energized. She was losing weight quickly, and it was motivating her to keep going. She received compliments from friends and family, which only boosted her confidence.

After a few months, Kayla had reached her goal weight. She was amazed by how much her body had changed and how much better she felt. She had lost over 20 pounds, and her skin was glowing. She also had a new-found appreciation for healthy eating and exercise.

The Scarsdale Diet had completely transformed Kayla's life. She felt happier, healthier, and more confident than she ever had before. She was grateful for the diet's effectiveness and was excited to maintain her new healthy lifestyle.

The Scarsdale Diet is a popular weight loss plan that was developed by Dr. Herman Tarnower in the 1970s. It is a low-carbohydrate, high-protein diet that is designed to help people lose weight quickly and effectively. The diet is based on the principle that by restricting carbohydrates, the body will burn stored fat for energy, leading to weight loss.

The Scarsdale Diet consists of two phases: the Initial Phase and the Maintenance Phase. During the Initial Phase, which lasts for two weeks, dieters are required to follow a strict meal plan that includes high-protein foods like chicken, fish, and eggs, as well as low-carb vegetables like spinach, broccoli, and asparagus. Dieters are also encouraged to drink plenty of water and avoid foods that are high in carbohydrates, such as bread, pasta, and rice.

After the Initial Phase, dieters can move on to the Maintenance Phase, which is designed to help them maintain their weight loss and prevent weight regain. During this phase, dieters can eat a wider range of foods and can even have occasional treats, like a small serving of chocolate or a glass of wine. However, they are still encouraged to limit their intake of carbohydrates and to focus on eating protein-rich foods.

Overall, the Scarsdale Diet is a effective weight loss plan that has helped many people shed excess pounds and improve their health. While it may be challenging to stick to the strict meal plan in the beginning,

the results can be well worth it in the
end.

Chapter one

The Scarsdale Diet's Scientific Basis

Dr. Herman Tarnower developed the well-known low-carb Scarsdale diet during the 1970s. The diet is predicated on the notion that consuming less carbohydrates while consuming more protein and fat might aid in weight reduction. This is due to the fact that the body produces sugar when carbs are ingested in excess, which might result in weight gain. The Scarsdale Diet urges the body to use fat for energy instead of carbohydrates by reducing carbohydrate consumption.

The Scarsdale Diet is a stringent eating regimen that calls for adhering to a set menu for two weeks, followed by one week of maintenance. Lean protein sources like chicken, fish, and eggs are prioritized in the diet, along with a daily amount of fruit and vegetables. Additionally, it promotes the use of wholesome fats like avocado and olive oil.

The diet has generated considerable debate since it is extremely low in calories and could not contain all the nutrients required for optimum health. The Scarsdale diet can, nevertheless, be beneficial for weight loss in the short term, according to certain research.

Overall, the Scarsdale Diet's scientific foundation is the notion that lowering carbohydrate intake might aid in weight reduction. Even though the diet may be successful for some individuals, it is crucial to speak with a healthcare professional before beginning any new eating plan.

The Scarsdale Diet GuidelinesThe "attack phase" and the "maintenance phase" are the two sections of the diet.

Dieters are only permitted to consume a limited number of items during the attack phase, including non-starchy greens like lettuce and spinach and lean proteins like chicken, fish, and turkey. Dieters may also have one serving of fruit each day and a small quantity of low-fat dairy products, such as plain yogurt or cottage cheese. Dieters are also advised to consume at least eight glasses of water each day in addition to these items.

Dieters should go on to the maintenance phase following the attack phase, which is supposed to last for two weeks. Dieters are permitted to consume a greater range of meals during this phase, including some complex carbs like whole grains and starchy vegetables. They are nevertheless urged to consume lean proteins and non-starchy veggies while limiting their consumption of high-fat items like fried dishes and red meat.

The Scarsdale Diet has drawn flak for being overly rigid and challenging to maintain over time. Concerns regarding its possible detrimental effects on health, such as a higher risk of heart disease and renal issues, have also been voiced by some specialists. Before beginning any weight-loss strategy, including the Scarsdale Diet, it is crucial to see a doctor.

The Rules of the Scarsdale Diet

The diet is divided into two phases: the "Attack Phase" and the "Maintenance Phase".

During the Attack Phase, dieters are allowed to eat only specific foods, including lean protein, such as chicken, fish, and turkey, and non-starchy vegetables, such as lettuce and spinach. Dieters are also allowed to have one serving of fruit per day, and a small amount of low-fat dairy, such as cottage cheese or plain yogurt. In addition to these foods, dieters are encouraged to drink at least eight glasses of water per day.

The Attack Phase is intended to last for two weeks, after which dieters move on to the Maintenance Phase. During this phase, dieters are allowed to eat a wider variety of foods, including some complex carbohydrates, such as whole grains and starchy vegetables. However, they are still encouraged to eat lean protein and non-non-starchy vegetables, and to limit their intake of high-fat foods, such as red meat and fried foods.

The Scarsdale Diet has been criticized for being too restrictive and difficult to follow long-term. Some experts have also raised concerns about its potential negative effects on health, including an increased risk of heart disease and kidney problems. It is important to talk to a doctor before starting any weight-loss plan, including the Scarsdale Diet.

What is the Scarsdale Diet?

The Scarsdale Diet is a weight loss plan that focuses on eating a high-protein, low-carbohydrate diet. The diet is based on a meal plan that includes specific foods and portions that are designed to help you lose weight quickly.

How does the Scarsdale Diet work?

The Scarsdale Diet works by restricting the types and amounts of carbohydrates that you eat. By limiting your intake of carbohydrates, your body is forced to burn stored fat for energy, which can lead to weight loss. Additionally, the high-protein content of the diet helps to keep you feeling full and satisfied.

How long does the Scarsdale Diet last?

The Scarsdale Diet is typically followed for a period of two weeks. After the initial two-week period, you can continue following the diet for as long as you like, or switch to a different weight loss plan.

What can you eat on the Scarsdale Diet?

The Scarsdale Diet allows you to eat a wide variety of foods, including lean proteins, non-starchy vegetables, and healthy fats. Some of the foods that are allowed on the diet include lean meats, fish, eggs, vegetables, and low-fat dairy products.

Can you exercise on the Scarsdale Diet?

Exercise is not required on the Scarsdale Diet, but it is recommended. Incorporating regular physical activity into your routine can help you to lose weight more quickly, and it can also have numerous health benefits. If you choose to exercise while following the Scarsdale Diet, be sure to talk to your doctor before starting a new workout routine.

Chapter two

The seven days meal plan

Day 1

Breakfast: Half a grapefruit, a slice of protein bread, and coffee or tea.

Lunch: Tuna salad made with canned tuna, mixed greens, cucumber, and lemon juice.

Snack: Carrot sticks with low-fat cottage cheese.

Dinner: Grilled chicken breast with steamed broccoli and a side salad.

Dessert: A small bowl of fresh strawberries.

Day 2

Breakfast: One hard-boiled egg, a slice of protein bread, and coffee or tea.

Lunch: Mixed greens salad with grilled chicken, tomatoes, and balsamic vinaigrette.

Snack: Celery sticks with a tablespoon of peanut butter.

Dinner: Grilled fish (such as salmon or cod) with roasted asparagus and a side salad.

Dessert: Sliced melon or a small portion of low-fat yogurt.

Day 3

Breakfast: Half a grapefruit, a slice of protein bread, and coffee or tea.

Lunch: Cottage cheese with sliced tomatoes and cucumbers.

Snack: A handful of almonds.

Dinner: Lean steak with steamed green beans and a side salad.

Dessert: Fresh berries with a dollop of low-fat whipped cream.

Day 4

Breakfast: One hard-boiled egg, a slice of protein bread, and coffee or tea.

Lunch: Grilled chicken or turkey breast with mixed greens and lemon juice dressing.

Snack: Sliced bell peppers with hummus.

Dinner: Baked fish with sautéed spinach and a side salad.

Dessert: Sugar-free gelatin with fresh fruit.

Note: Remember to stay hydrated throughout the diet by drinking water or unsweetened beverages.

Day 5

Breakfast: Half of a grapefruit, a slice of protein bread, and black coffee or tea.

Lunch: Egg salad made with hard-boiled eggs, mixed with a little mayonnaise, and served on lettuce leaves.

Dinner: Baked or broiled fish, steamed vegetables (green beans, bell peppers, or cabbage), and a green salad with lemon juice.

Snack: Raw radishes or cucumber slices.

Note: Remember to drink plenty of water throughout the day and avoid all oils, fats, and added sugars while following the Scarsdale Diet.

Sample Recipes:

Grilled Lemon Chicken:

Ingredients:

- 4 skinless, boneless chicken breasts
- Juice of 1 lemon
- Salt and pepper to taste

Instructions:

- Preheat the grill to medium-high heat.

- Season the chicken breasts with salt, pepper, and lemon juice.

- Grill the chicken for about 6-8 minutes on each side or until cooked through.

- Serve with steamed vegetables and a green salad.

Tuna and White Bean Salad:
Ingredients:

- 1 can water-packed tuna, drained
- 1 can white beans, drained and rinsed
- 1/2 red onion, diced
- Juice of 1 lemon
- Salt and pepper to taste
- Fresh parsley for garnish (optional)

Instructions:

- In a bowl, combine the tuna, white beans, diced red onion, lemon juice, salt, and pepper.

- Mix well to combine all the ingredients.

- Garnish with fresh parsley if desired.

- Serve on a bed of lettuce or as a filling for protein bread.

Steamed Vegetables Medley:
Ingredients:

- Assorted vegetables of your choice (broccoli florets, cauliflower florets, and sliced carrots)
- Salt to taste
- Lemon juice for drizzling

Instructions:

- Steam the vegetables until tender but still crisp.
- Season with salt and drizzle with lemon juice.
- Toss gently to combine.

Serve as a side dish with your main protein source.

7 Tips and Tricks for Sticking to the 7 Scarsdale Diet

Scarsdale diet

It is known for its fast weight loss results, but can be challenging to stick to due to its strict meal plan. Here are a few tips and tricks for sticking to the 7 Scarsdale Diet:

1. Plan ahead: Before starting the diet, make a meal plan for the week and shop for all the necessary ingredients. This will help you stay on track and avoid making impulsive food choices.

2. Stay hydrated: Drink plenty of water throughout the day to help keep your body hydrated and to curb hunger.

3. Don't skip meals: The Scarsdale Diet involves eating small, frequent meals throughout the day. Skipping meals can cause you to become overly hungry, which can lead to overeating or making poor food choices.

4. Stay motivated: It can be easy to lose motivation when following a strict diet. Find ways to stay motivated, such as keeping a food journal, setting small goals, or seeking support from friends or a support group.

5. Be prepared for challenges: There will inevitably be challenges when sticking to any diet, and the Scarsdale Diet is no exception. Be prepared for these challenges and have a plan in place for how to overcome them. For example, if you are going to a social event where there will be unhealthy food, plan to bring your own healthy option or choose the healthiest options available.

6. Be consistent: Consistency is key when it comes to any diet. Stick to the meal plan and don't give up, even if you have a bad day or slip up. It's

important to remember that weight loss is a journey and it's normal to have setbacks along the way.

7. Consult a healthcare professional: Before starting the Scarsdale Diet or any other diet, it's important to consult with a healthcare professional to ensure it is safe and appropriate for you. A healthcare professional can also provide guidance and support to help you stick to the diet and achieve your weight loss goals.

The Scarsdale Diet recommends eating three meals a day, with snacks in between if needed. Here are some snack ideas for the first seven days of the diet.

Cottage cheese with sliced tomato

Mix half cup of low-fat cottage cheese with one sliced tomato. This snack is high in protein and low in carbohydrates.

Hard-boiled egg with a slice of turkey

Hard-boil one egg and slice it in half. Serve with a slice of turkey for added protein and flavor.

Apple slices with almond butter

Slice one apple and spread 1 tablespoon of almond butter on top. This snack is sweet and satisfying, and it provides healthy fats and protein.

Raw vegetables with hummus

Cut up a variety of raw vegetables, such as carrots, celery, and bell peppers. Serve with two tablespoons of hummus for added flavor and protein.

Greek yogurt with berries

Mix half cup of Greek yogurt with a handful of berries. This snack is high in protein and low in carbohydrates.

Turkey roll-up

Take one slice of turkey and roll it up with a slice of cheese and a lettuce leaf. This snack is satisfying and portable.

Edamame

Steam a cup of edamame and sprinkle it with a pinch of sea salt. This snack is high in protein and fiber.

Remember to drink plenty of water throughout the day to stay hydrated and support your weight loss efforts. The Scarsdale Diet recommends drinking at least eight glasses of water a day.

One component of the diet is to incorporate smoothies into your daily routine. Below are seven smoothie recipes that you can try as part of the Scarsdale diet:

- **Spinach and Strawberry Smoothie**

Combine one cup of baby spinach, one cup of sliced strawberries, half cup of low-fat yogurt, and half cup of ice in a blender. Blend until smooth and enjoy.

- **Blueberry and Banana Smoothie**

Combine one cup of frozen blueberries, one frozen banana, half cup of unsweetened almond milk, and half cup of ice in a blender. Blend until smooth and enjoy.

- **Mango and Peach Smoothie**

Combine one cup of frozen mango chunks, one cup of frozen peaches, one cup of low-fat yogurt, and half cup of ice in a blender. Blend until smooth and enjoy.

- **Raspberry and Blackberry Smoothie**

Combine one cup of frozen raspberries, one cup of frozen blackberries, half cup of unsweetened almond milk, and half cup of ice in a blender. Blend until smooth and enjoy.

- **Pineapple and Coconut Smoothie**

Combine one cup of frozen pineapple chunks, half cup of unsweetened coconut milk, half cup of low-fat yogurt, and half cup of ice in a blender. Blend until smooth and enjoy.

- **Watermelon and Mint Smoothie**

Combine one cup of cubed watermelon, one fourth cup of fresh mint leaves, half cup of low-fat yogurt, and half cup of ice in a blender. Blend until smooth and enjoy.

- **Cucumber and Lime Smoothie**

Combine one cup of sliced cucumber, half cup of low-fat yogurt,One tablespoon of lime juice, and half cup of ice in a blender. Blend until smooth and enjoy.

Remember to consult with your doctor before starting any new diet or

exercise plan, including the Scarsdale
diet.

Chapter three

Maintenance and Long-term Weight Loss with the Scarsdale Diet

The Scarsdale Diet is a popular weight loss program that has been around since the 1970s. It is a low-carbohydrate, high-protein diet that is designed to help people lose weight quickly. The diet is divided into two phases: the initial weight loss phase, during which people can expect to lose up to 20 pounds in 14 days, and the maintenance phase, which is designed to help people keep the weight off in the long term.

During the initial weight loss phase of the Scarsdale Diet, people are encouraged to eat a high-protein, low-carbohydrate diet that is rich in lean meats, fish, and non-starchy vegetables. The diet includes specific meal plans and recipes, and emphasizes the importance of regular exercise.

Once people have reached their target weight, they enter the maintenance phase of the Scarsdale Diet. This phase is designed to help people maintain their weight loss in the long term. The maintenance phase includes a number of strategies to help people keep the weight off, including:

- Continuing to eat a balanced diet that is low in carbohydrates and high in protein
- Incorporating regular exercise into their daily routine
- Monitoring their weight and making adjustments to their diet and exercise habits as needed

One of the key challenges of the Scarsdale Diet is sticking to it in the long term. The diet can be difficult to maintain because it is so restrictive, and many people find it hard to stick to the strict meal plans and recipes.

It is important to be patient and to make gradual changes to the diet in order to avoid feeling overwhelmed or deprived. By making these changes and sticking to a healthy lifestyle, it is possible to achieve long-term weight loss success with the Scarsdale Diet.

Conclusion

After researching and learning about the Scarsdale Diet, it is clear that this is a low-carbohydrate and low-fat diet that focuses on lean protein and non-starchy vegetables. The diet is structured and provides specific meal plans and guidelines to follow.

One of the main benefits of the Scarsdale Diet is that it promotes rapid weight loss and can help individuals reach their weight loss goals quickly. However, it is important to note that this diet may not be sustainable for long-term weight maintenance and may require individuals to make significant changes to their eating habits.

In conclusion, starting the Scarsdale Diet may be a good option for individuals who are looking for a structured and rapid weight loss plan. However, it is important to consult with a healthcare professional before starting any new diet and to carefully consider the potential drawbacks and challenges of this diet.

As next steps, individuals interested in starting the Scarsdale Diet should speak with a healthcare professional and review the meal plans and guidelines provided by the diet. It may also be helpful to reach out to others who have successfully completed the Scarsdale Diet and seek their advice and support.